The 10-Day 'At-Home' Colon Cleansing Formula

Detoxify Your Body, Lose Weight, Get Healthy & Transform Your Life Volume 1

ROBERT DAVE JOHNSTON

Published by:

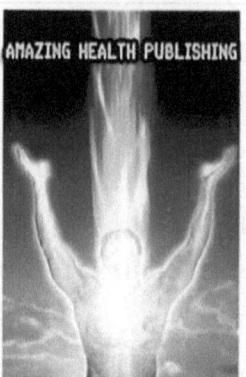

If you are interested in reading the next volume,
follow Rob on Twitter @RobDaveJohnston

Copyright

Disclaimer & Legal Notices

The health-related information and suggestions contained in any of the books or written material mentioned above are based on the research, experience and opinions of the Author and other contributors. Nothing herein should be misinterpreted as actual medical advice, such as one would obtain from a Physician, or as advice for self-diagnosis or as any manner of prescription for self-treatment.

Neither is any information herein to be considered a particular or general cure for any ailment, disease or other health issue. The material contained within is offered strictly and solely for the purpose of providing Holistic health education to the general public. Persons with any health condition should consult a medical professional before entering this or any fasting, weight loss, detoxification or health related program.

Even if you suffer from no known illness, we recommend that you seek medical advice before starting any fasting, weight loss and/or detoxification program, and before choosing to follow any advice given this book. For any products or services mentioned or suggested in this book, you should read all packaging and instructions, as no substance, natural or drug, can be guaranteed to work in everyone.

Information and statements regarding dietary supplements, products or services mentioned in this book many not have been evaluated by the Food and Drug Administration and are not intended to diagnose, treat, cure, or prevent any disease. Never disregard or delay in seeking professional medical advice because of something you have read in this book.

Nothing that you read in this book should be regarded as medical or health advice. If you do anything recommended in this book, without the supervision of a licensed medical doctor, you do so at your own risk. Not recommended for persons with any health related condition unless supervised by a qualified health practitioner.

Because there is always some risk involved in any health-related program, the Author, Publisher and contributors assume no responsibility for any adverse effects or consequences resulting from the use of any suggested preparations or procedures described in any of the books or other written materials associated with the website FitnessThroughFasting.com. The author reserves the right to alter and update his opinions based on new conditions at any time.

Dedication

This series of books are dedicated to my mother Sonia Noemi, without whom I would not even be alive today. I love you mom. Thank you for never losing faith in me and supporting me, even when everything seemed hopeless and everyone else had given up on me. I owe you everything. I could collect all of the precious stones on this earth and lay them on your lap, and even still, I would not even come close to giving back to you all that you have given me.

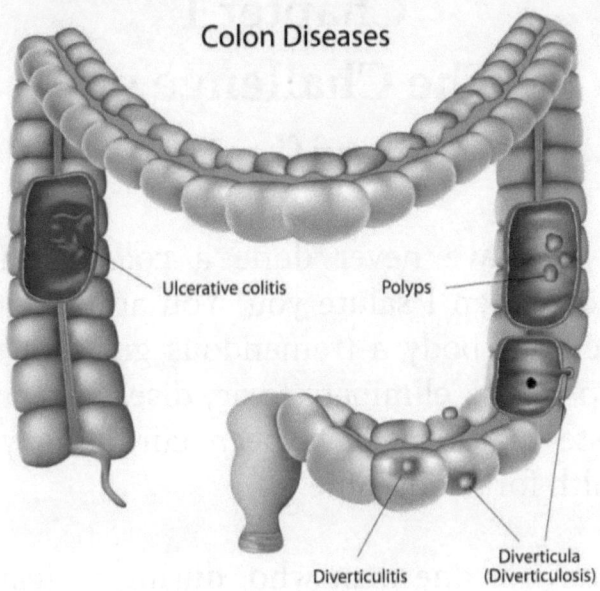

Colon Diseases

Ulcerative colitis   Polyps

Diverticulitis   Diverticula (Diverticulosis)

"By picking up this book, you are making drastic changes in your life. Change requires vision, sacrifice and determination. There is, however, something you must keep very clear in your mind: *"The benefits of sticking to your guns and following through with this process are monumental and life-changing."*

Chapter 1
The Challenge of Detoxification

If you have never done a colon cleanse before, then I salute you: You are about to give your body a tremendous gift that will help you to eliminate toxic, disease-causing waste that may have been curtailing your health for a long time.

I know of one man who, during a cleanse, eliminated several pounds of rotten, undigested meat from his colon. And, to be sure, examples like that abound. In this book, I am going to give you a simple and straightforward method to achieve ultimate colon cleansing, from the comfort of your own home. I struggled with liver and colon toxicity for many years; in fact, at one point it got so bad that I thought my days were numbered. But by being consistent as well as patient, I was able to turn my health around, and that has happened to a great extent thanks to the colon cleansing remedy presented here. I was far gone physically; a morbidly obese, self-destructive basket case. If this can work for someone like me (*who reached low bottoms of food addiction and obesity*), then by all means I believe that it will do wonders for you as well.

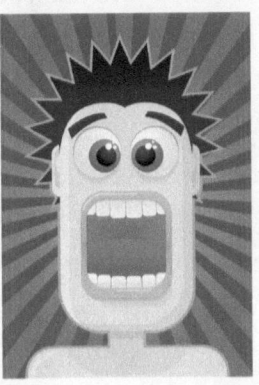

Rectal Phobia

I know that any procedure involving the rectum will never be on anyone's *Top 10* list of '*Most Wanted.*' It took me years to let go of my prejudice against colon cleansing; that is, until I reached a point of desperation and became willing to do it – **FOR MYSELF**. If you feel resistant to colon cleansing because it involves (more than usual) anal discharging and feces, please get over it. How would your house be if you put the trash on bags but never took them out? Can you imagine the stench, cockroaches and filth that would result? The same happens with our bodies.

When the colon is strained from poor and/or excessive eating, a lot of the debris that is supposed to go out lingers, rotting and intoxicating the bloodstream, which, in turn, adversely affects the functioning of vital organs – even the brain. If you can see it from that perspective, it will be easier to get through the resistance. I'm certain that you do not want toxic trash circulating around your body creating havoc. Once you take action, you will begin to see colon cleansing in a whole new light.

Persistence and Patience

And I am very glad that I did. Within a few days of my first cleanse, I started to feel lighter, more energized and my mood swings, which had become very volatile and painful, began to stabilize. The key is persistence and patience. Persistence in taking the action, and patience in allowing the body to do what it does *at its pace.* I say this because many people write to tell me that, "*they did a colon cleanse and nothing came out.*" Well, imagine if a soft piece of clay is permitted to harden and become as tough as a rock. How many times will you have to pound the rock with a pick before it finally comes apart? The same is the case with our bodies.

If you have eaten poorly for a long time, or even if you haven't, chances are that you will need to be patient and try, try again if the initial cleansing doesn't produce the desired results.

Please... I am begging you: **Take the action**, but be patient and good to your body. It will **ALWAYS** produce the outcomes you desire, IF you are long-suffering and unrelenting.

And by no means increase the dosages in this colon cleanse formula, even if at first you do not see much discharge.

Keep working at it, follow my instructions, and – eventually- it will happen. That has been my experience over the years, and I am certain that you, too, will achieve great things through this type of cleanse.

Home Remedy Vs. Cleansing Kits

I have put this book together so that it is short and to-the-point. I give you a list of ingredients that you will need for the "*at-home*" cleansing remedy.

If you do not have time to prepare these home remedies, or if you simply do not wish to delve into the matter that deeply, I have also presented a kit alternative.

However, I strongly encourage you to take the time and learn to prepare the home remedy.

Having that type of holistic knowledge (*knowing how to detox your body*) is invaluable. No matter where you may find yourself, you will be able to put together a home colon-cleanse remedy.

The ingredients are available at your local supermarket, health food store or herb/produce vendor. I buy a lot of them online at amazon.com.

Note: None of what we are doing here is easy. You are making drastic changes in your life. Change requires vision, sacrifice and determination. There is, however, something you must keep very clear in your mind:

"The benefits of sticking to your guns and following through with this process are monumental and life-changing".

Clarify and expand your goals. Write in a journal what your goals are in relation to your health. Remind yourself **DAILY** exactly why you want to detoxify and improve your health.

You will feel great pride and self-esteem when following through until you accomplish your goals. These positive feelings will last much longer than the piece of chocolate cake you are reaching for. Now is the time! Stop giving up and returning to your old ways. Remember:

**A minute on the lips,
forever on the hips!**

Chapter 2
Constipation

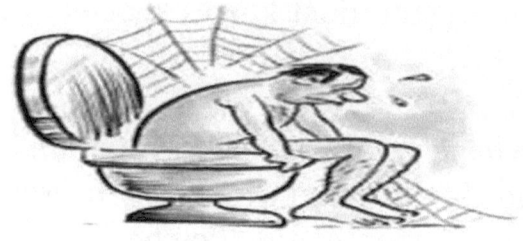

There is an old saying that you have to: *"exhale before you can inhale"*. Put another way, it is necessary to empty before one can fill. The same applies to the colon. You have to drain what is inside before you can nourish. You can eat all the health-food in the world, but if your colon is clogged and polluted, the benefit will be paltry. That is the "why" of colon cleansing.

One of the most frequent problems people experience today is constipation. A constipated system is one in which the transition time of toxic waste is slow. The longer the "*transit time*," the longer the toxic matter sits in the bowel. This allows the waste to putrefy, ferment and – even worse - be reabsorbed into the blood stream.

The longer your body has putrefying food in the intestines, the greater the risk of developing disease.

Did you know? -> Even if you have one bowel movement per day, you could still have several meals worth of waste-matter in your colon! I don't know about you, but that does **NOT** sound very pleasant.

Bowel movements are the basis of human health. If you don't have at least **ONE** bowel movement per day, then you are probably walking towards disease. Anatomically-speaking, the human body has not changed much over the past millennia. But, the food that we eat has. Refined sugar, white flour, hormone/antibiotic-filled meats and saturated fats have literally taken over the daily diet - especially in the US.

This type of highly-processed food causes great harm to the digestive system. It also keeps the body addicted. I just finished a great book called *"The End of Overeating"* by Dr. David Kessler. In it, he goes into great detail in his coverage of the fast food industry and the American diet. I encourage you to read it. If your diet has been less than optimum, then all congestion and toxins must be removed.

This begins with colon cleansing, and here's the bottom line: One of the greatest challenges our bodies face is the effective removal of wastes and toxins. As the colon becomes impacted with putrefied waste, its shape can stretch like a balloon and develop Diverticulitis – a dangerous condition of inflammation which can become infected. In advanced cases, prolonged constipation and straining could even lead to Rectal Prolapse.

Chapter 3
Is Your Colon Healthy?

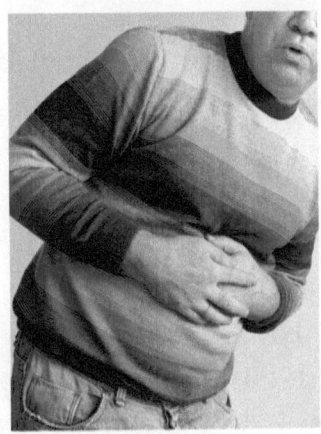

If you are experiencing any of the symptoms listed below, then your digestive system is probably **NOT** in the best of health. You may have an unhealthy colon if you:

* **Have infrequent bowel movements or very small amounts**. Small pellet-shaped stools are a common indication that something is wrong.

***Need to strain to eliminate.** The toilet is no place to get an "abdominal workout". Effortless and quick bowel movements are key signs of a healthy colon.

* Require a substantial amount of time to go. If you have a 500-page novel next to the toilet as opposed to the newspaper, that may be a clue!

When I visited a friend recently and saw a copy of *"War and Peace"* in the bathroom, I knew he needed a colon cleanse.

This book will focus on an *"at-home"* colon cleansing system I learned years ago when I struggled with a toxic liver. It is very powerful and can be used any time your digestion is sluggish, you feel heavy, congested or lethargic - or when you are coming down with a cold.

Headaches, bad breath, white coat on the tongue, bloating and constant flatulence are all indicators that it is time for a colon cleanse.

So keep this book handy. You can use it in the future or pass it on to a loved-one who may need it!

Important Reminder

Constipation and other bowel disorders can be a sign of a serious condition. If you find that you do not have a bowel movement in spite of this cleanse, then I strongly encourage you to see your doctor at once. A variety of diseases can cause irregularity of the bowels. Disease often begins with a toxic bowel. Fewer bowel movements harbor a potentially-fertile breeding ground for sickness. Infrequent or poor quality bowel movements over an extended period of time can be hazardous to your health.

LIKEWISE,

Use Common Sense! **Discontinue this colon-cleanse if you experience persistent diarrhea for longer than two days.** Drink at least half-a-gallon of water daily while on this cleanse. If you are more than 20 pounds overweight, as much as three days of diarrhea may be normal, especially if you have never done a cleanse before. If you are <u>NOT</u> overweight, then you must be vigilant and follow your instinct when doing this type of cleanse.

Chapter 4
Pre-Cleanse Preparation

If you have been eating poorly and/or excessively, your colon cleansing efforts will go a lot further if you prepare your body. And that means removing from your diet any and all junk, greasy and sugary foods that you are accustomed to eating. The removal of these toxic foods will send your body into ultimate detoxification mode, and it will work hard on your behalf to eliminate the filth that keeps you from experiencing optimal health and wellness.

Of course, usual offenders that must be eliminated (*at least during the ten-day colon cleanse*) are sugars, starches (*enriched flour*) and saturated fats.

These include but are not limited to pastries, candy, white rice, white bread, soda pops, butter, frying oil, cheeseburgers, pizza, etc...For further guidance, here is a list of *'banned foods.'* Stay away from then during the ten-day cleanse.

I'd love it if you stayed away from them permanently, as your health, energy and overall wellness would shoot off the charts if you did. However, for the sake of this immediate cleanse, you are to abstain from all of the foods listed below during the 10-day period.

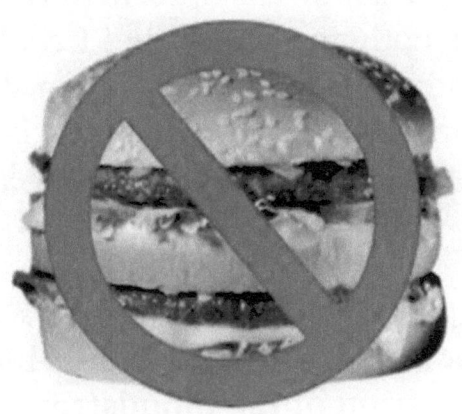

Banned Foods

*Salt - you get plenty of it from the foods that you eat. When I first started my diet years ago, I was kind of shocked to see that salt was banned. I spoke against it actually. I have come to realize that the foods we eat all have sodium, and that a healthy adult really has no need for 'salt' except to make the food taste better.

In addition, when I stopped using salt, I immediately dropped like 15 pounds. It was mostly water weight, but it showed me that I was retaining a <u>LOT</u> of liquids, and that was greatly due to my abuse of salt and seasonings.

* **Sugar** - absolute trash, toxic to the body... good for nothing - stay away! I could write pages and pages about sugar. I am sure that you yourself can admit that this is one of our greatest (*if not our greatest*) enemy. I mean it. Enemy.

Any prolonged return to sugar will, sooner or later, result in full-blown intoxication of the bloodstream and digestive system.

I don't kid myself by thinking that "I'm cured." I still am susceptible to sugar and to binging. What keeps me free and clean is **NOT** to put sugar into my body... period.

I can't draw the same conclusion for you, but I am certain that you probably have your own stories to tell about sugar and how it has affected your weight, life and health.

* **Fried Foods** - Absolute filthy grease fest that leads to obesity and other diseases.

* **Cheese** - Cheese is great but it has way too much fat. For the time being, steer clear. Later on, once you finish the cleanse, you will be able to have treats from time to time. So don't let the mind start telling you that your 'life is over' because you can't eat this or that. Just tell the mind to shut up and keep moving forward. Works like a charm for me.

* **Dairy Products** - dairy has a lot of fat, is high in sugar content and has been known to cause digestive system inflammation. But I'm not totally heartless. Stick to non-fat milk, how's that? Anything above non-fat is banned.

* **Red Meat** - I personally don't have anything against red meat. In fact, I have been known to eat a piece of meat on rare occasion. Right now, we are banning it because it has a lot of fat, and because I want your digestive system to be given easy food to digest. Later on you can have a piece of meat here and there if you want. Right now... it's banned.

* **Alcohol** - Alcohol is packed with empty calories. Calories with **ZERO** nutritional value. And booze turns to sugar. Bad all over. If you drink frequently, cut it down to a minimum. You're doing this for your health and to reach a goal that is important to **YOU**. If you have to go a few days without drinking, your arm is not going to fall off. You'll live. A cup of wine with dinner is fine, but nothing more than that at this juncture.

* **Butter or Margarine** - As they say in New York, "Forget about it!!!" Butter and margarine are pure fat and we don't want it.

* **Fruit Juices** - If you read the label of most orange juice brands, you will see that the sugar content is through the roof. Yes, it is natural sugar, but sugar nonetheless.

You can have one glass of juice in the morning, but you need to water it down 50/50. Drinking straight juice at this phase is basically like injecting blubber directly into your belly. Stay away. Drink veggie juice instead...but make sure that it is the low sodium veggie juice.

*White Enriched Bread - That stuff is like dropping a ball of cement into the stomach. White flour, doughy garbage really is terrible for human health. I was going to ban all breads, but I remembered that the Ezekiel brand (*green bag*) is actually very good. You can eat one slice here and there as partial replacement to your carbohydrate servings. We'll get into all of that in just a minute.

*Junk Food of ANY Kind - I think that it definitely goes without saying that junk food is out. And not just out for a little while.

Hopefully, it is out of your life for good. That crap is like wearing a ball and chain. It enslaves us to cravings that are never satisfied and only get stronger and more violent.

Foods to Limit List:

*Fruits (Stick To Strawberries or Cantaloupe)
* Tomatoes
* Peas or Corn
* Olive Oil

Starting immediately, eliminate <u>ALL</u> of these foods and beverages from your diet... period.

This is the beginning of the process. For now, continue to eat whatever else you have been eating **EXCEPT** for the foods that are listed above. I want you to take a full step forward and discontinue eating any and all junk. That's the whole point of our work together, right? To help you achieve measurable improvements in your health. So cut it all out. Do not eat <u>even a little</u> of them anymore. I mean <u>Nothing</u>, <u>No More</u>, <u>Finito</u>, <u>Nada</u>!

You are taking the <u>monumental</u> step of removing **ALL** toxic foods from your diet. I use the word *'monumental'* because, in truth, you are now in the minority. The majority of people live their whole lives and **NEVER** confront their eating behaviors as you are now doing.

And since you won't be dumping more and more crap into your belly, the colon cleansing remedy will be able to focus on the breakdown and discharge of existing debris.

Chapter 5
Eat Six Times Daily

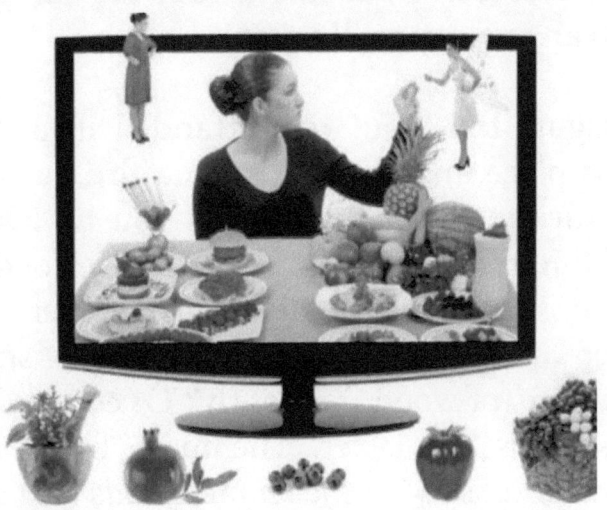

Eating smaller meals with greater frequency, totaling six meals per day, is one of the strategies that helped me to expel the most intestinal debris through colon cleansing. I would strongly encourage you to observe the banned foods list during the 10-day colon cleanse, as well as change your eating structure to one of six smaller meals.

This method will accelerate your metabolism, meaning that the body can process and expel toxins faster and more efficiently. But, don't worry... this doesn't have to be hard.

The six-meals-per-day structure includes breakfast, mid-morning snack, lunch, mid-afternoon snack, dinner and evening snack. The metabolism is like a fire. Let me give you an analogy to illustrate.

Imagine that you were stranded in a very cold place and need to keep a fire burning to survive the night. Would you be better off dumping a huge amount of firewood at once, or would the fire burn longer and keep you warmer if you added small amounts of wood frequently? Of course, the answer is the latter. The more frequently you eat (*observing the banned foods list*), the better you will feel and the more energy you will have.

Consequently, the metabolism will work evenly and continuously, which results in faster weight loss and elimination of toxins.

Having larger meals with less frequency is like dumping a large amount of wood into the fire. You will get one heck of blaze initially, but it will die out sooner and not provide as much heat (*energy*) as it would if you added wood more sparingly.

This is what causes the monster cravings that keep people trapped in binging and overeating for years. If you want to disconnect the cravings and succeed in your colon cleansing, eat more frequently.

To help you see how this works, here is a sample menu from a typical day in my life:

Sample Menu

Breakfast 8:00 AM

1 Cup of Oatmeal with 1 Cup Skim Milk, a Handful of Raisins or Plums
Three Egg Whites mixed with, 3 OZ Ground Turkey
1 Cup of Green Tea with Stevia

Mid-Morning Snack 10AM

1 Apple or Pear Mixed With One Cup of Nonfat Yogurt (Plain)
OR, ONE Apple, Pear, Banana or Other Fruit

Lunch - Noon

Big salad with lettuce, tomato and other veggies you may like. For dressing, use olive oil (no more than 1 teaspoon) and balsamic vinegar.
1 Envelope of Low-Sodium Tuna
1 4OZ Baked Potato or Sweet Potato

Mid-Afternoon Snack 3PM

Same as before - I usually have a piece of fruit mixed with yogurt. At this time in the afternoon, I also drink another cup of green tea. Green tea has energy-boosting and body-heating properties. It will help to give you a pep as well as calm hunger pangs. In addition to green tea, seltzer water (*sparkling water/club soda*) is great to navigate hunger.

Dinner - 6PM

Six-to-eight ounces of chicken, fish or ground turkey (I like to make turkey patties)
Large salad as the one eaten for lunch
Steamed Broccoli, Cauliflower and Carrots (*most supermarkets have prepackaged*

vegetable combinations that are ready to steam and eat).
4OZ Baked Potato or Sweet Potato OR 4OZ of Whole Wheat or Whole Grain Pasta OR 4 OZ of Brown Rice

Evening Snack - 8PM

Big salad with 3OZ Chicken, Fish or Ground Turkey - No carbohydrates.
A piece of fruit with Non-fat Yogurt
Cup of Chamomile Tea - Chamomile tea is great to drink at night because it will help soothe hunger as well as calm you and get you ready for bed.

You should not eat anything at least two hours prior to turning in. Sometimes I also take one 500 mg tablet of Tryptophan at night to help me sleep.

Tryptophan is an awesome amino acid that helps to stabilize mood. At this point I'm done eating for the day and drink only water until 8AM the following morning.

Again -> **NEVER EAT FOR THE LAST TWO HOURS BEFORE YOU GO TO BED**.

Do you ingest a large portion of your daily calories a few hours before bedtime?

When your body is at rest, all of your metabolic processes slow down so you don't burn as many calories as you would during the day while you are actively moving around. When you eat large portions of food shortly before you go to bed, many of those calories are going to be stored as fat.

Unfortunately, some people eat very few calories all day long, then gulp down a large dinner – and then munch on snacks all evening before they go to bed! Throughout the day they may have ingested 500 to 700 calories, and then 2,000 to 3,000 calories right before they go to bed. Bad idea! Tape your mouth shut if you have to. But eat no more!

Chapter 6
Home Colon Cleansing

Alright, let's take a look at the ingredients you will need to prepare your home colon cleansing formula. Each of the ingredients listed below are the very same that I use to prepare my own colon cleansing remedy. After years of frequent colon cleansings, even with at-home colonic kits, these products are the ones that produce the very best results. You can order them online and they should arrive in roughly two days.

Alternatively, you can browse for them in your local health food store or supermarket. I like Amazon because, in 99% of the cases, the prices are notably lower, and the shipping is fast. At the bottom of the list you will note that I mention the Lifiber colon cleansing kit as an alternative. As I said earlier, go with the kit only if you absolutely, positively do not have the time or disposition to prepare the remedy.

My suggestion is that you definitely use the remedy, get acquainted with it and master it. You don't know if a kit will be around at a time of need, while the basic ingredients in the remedy are easily found pretty much everywhere. Once you get comfortable preparing the remedy and **SEE** the amazing results, there's no doubt that this kind of holistic medicine will stay in your family for the long-term.

Colon Cleanse Formula Ingredients

Organic Apple Juice - Apple juice helps the body fight-off bad cholesterol while enhancing cardiovascular health. It also combats constipation, cleans the liver and kidneys and is known to boost intestinal/colon health.

Apple Cider Vinegar - Diminishes sinus infections, effectively treats skin conditions such as acne, boosts the immune system, speeds-up the metabolism and promotes weight loss.

Helps to improve digestion and relieves constipation, can help fight-off the development of bladder stones and urinary tract infections.

It also relieves symptoms associated with gout and arthritis.

Aloe Vera Juice (<u>NOT</u> "Drink") Aids digestion, promotes weight loss, decreases blood sugar levels, boosts the immune system.

Psyllium Husk Powder (*Preferably Unflavored*) - Constipation Relief. Psyllium Husk Powder is a bulk laxative highly effective in the treatment of constipation.

When ingested, the powder absorbs water and turns into a gelatinous ball inside the digestive system. As it expands, jellylike ball pushes waste products out of the colon by force, triggering what can often be massive bowel movements.

Furthermore, Psyllium has lubricating properties which facilitate the passage of stool, thus reducing pain in cases of chronic hemorrhoids or colitis. Psyllium also treats diarrhea by absorbing extra water in the digestive tract and helping to make stools firm.

Cascara Sagrada -> Cascara Sagrada is a herbal laxative which is retrieved from the reddish bark of the Pacific Northwest native three, Rhamnus purshiana.

Liquid Chlorophyll - helps the body to flush out toxic heavy metals such as mercury. Liquid Chlorophyll assists in the removal of germs as well as thwarts the growth of new ones. Boosts digestive system functions.

Average Cost of This Remedy -> $50

OR, <u>ONE, MAYBE TWO</u> LiFiber Colon Detox Kits @ app. $65.95 each. Of the few 'cleansing kits' that I've used over the years, this LiFiber is, by far, the strongest and most complete. If you choose to go this path, make sure to read the instructions on the box before starting. Overall, the Lifiber would be taken at night just like the remedy.

The difference here is that all you need to add is water. It isn't necessary to mix various ingredients as is the case with the traditional remedy.

Still, I vote in favor of the remedy because it places at your fingertips a very powerful remedy that will always get the job done. It may seem like a drudgery at first to mix this with that and that.

But once you get used to it, you will hopefully come to love it as much as I do.

*I Recommend That You Do This 10-Day Colon Cleanse Again in <u>TWO</u> Months as Follow up, and Then At least Once Annually Thereafter.

Chapter 7
Preparing the Remedy

Once you have purchased all of the items, make some room in the kitchen counter so that you can work, setting aside any appliances or other objects that will get in the way. Bottom line: give yourself plenty of counter space. Get a used towel, one that you aren't particularly fond of, and lay it on top of the counter. Take out all of the ingredients and line them up around the towel. In addition, you will need a 16-ounce plastic or glass cup in which to mix the ingredients. Some people prefer to wear gloves when preparing these remedies; that's left totally to your discretion.

Add into the 16-ounce cup:

.

•1 heaping teaspoon Psyllium Husk Powder - (preferably unflavored)

•1/2 cup organic, unfiltered (*preferably raw or unpasteurized*) apple juice – if you cannot find raw apple juice, then pasteurized is acceptable if you add a tablespoon of Apple Cider Vinegar.

•2 tablespoons Chlorophyll.

•2 capsules of Cascara Sagrada - herbal laxative. Simply open the capsule and dump the brownish powder into the glass.

•2 tablespoons Aloe Vera Juice – make sure to get juice, not drink. Aloe Vera drinks are mostly water and <u>NOT</u> what we are looking for here.

•A 12-ounce glass of water.

Mix vigorously for 30 seconds and down the hatch! Drink the colon-cleansing formula nightly **TWO** hours before going to bed. Make sure to drink it right-away after you mix it because

Psyllium bulks up quickly. After you drink the first glass, there will nearly-always be residue.

Refill the glass with water, stir the contents and drink up until <u>**ALL**</u> of the contents are gone. Do this every night for the next <u>**TEN**</u> days.

Belly Massage

Many times, the intestinal debris in our bodies is very hard and stubborn, not wanting to let go of the walls of the colon. Spend as much time as possible massaging your stomach with both hands –covering the left, right, bottom and upper parts of the abdomen. Pay close attention to your liver. Play some music and let it sink in; visualize toxins, parasites and hardened fecal matter being expelled from your body.

Take as much time as needed in this process. I once had a female friend step on my stomach and move her foot all around the belly. She didn't put ALL of her weight on my stomach; just enough to exert some pressure. And, to my amazement, five minutes later I was sprinting to the toilet and ended up expelling a huge, black rock of debris that I'm certain had been inside of me for years. Really, really work it!

For some people with large levels of toxicity, the evacuation process can be dramatic and almost immediate. If that is the case for you, go ahead and eliminate.

You may feel cramps in your stomach and some abdomen pain. This is fairly normal for most people. Make sure to look at the discharge once you are done. What color is it? Is it really dark or even black? If so, then it is likely that you are making good progress. If at any time you see blood in the stool, stop the cleanse immediately and go see your doctor at once!

Chapter 8
Detox Symptoms

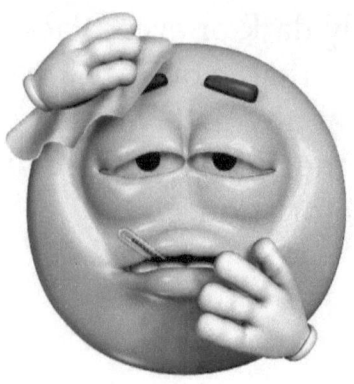

Changing your eating habits in the way that I have described is **<u>HUGE</u>**. It will cause your body to enter a process of deep detoxification. This will result in temporary discomfort while the body purges itself of toxins.

The good news is that, while you may not feel it, the symptoms indicate that you are getting healthier and stronger.

Keep that in mind as you traverse this phase of the program. Here are the primary symptoms that you can expect to experience.

Headaches – This one is especially marked for coffee drinkers, but is also the case for persons who consume large amounts of sugar and alcohol. This symptom can really take a person out of commission. A lot of my colleagues call me a heretic for saying this, but if you need to take a couple of ibuprofen tablets to ease the pain, then so be it.

Usually two tablets will do the trick. But don't take more than four daily. You may need to go through a little pain and discomfort. The good news is that headaches rarely last more than 72 hours, if that.

Dizziness – The body is not used to being deprived of eating whatever it wants and will go through dizzy spells, particularly during the first 11 days. The best solution for dizziness is to move slowly and get as much rest as your daily schedule allows.

Difficulty Performing Basic Tasks – Since you aren't consuming solid food, it will take some time for the body to adjust. You will more than likely feel very weak and may have trouble getting around - particularly during the first 10-14 days.

If you slow down and work on focusing on the individual tasks you are performing, this symptom can be overcome. It is important for you to realize that your body is going through a transition. You must move slowly and not try to push yourself too hard. You may not be able to function at the same capacity as you are accustomed. Fine. Slow down and give the body time to work on your behalf.

Weakness means that you need to be extra careful when walking around, and especially when getting up from a sitting position.

Avoid harsh and/or abrupt movements

Move slowly, watch your step closely and always have something that you can hang on to if you suddenly feel like you are fainting. This is good advice.

One time I totally hit the deck because I got up to quickly from a chair. I missed the corner of the wall by centimeters, but still hit myself quite hard on the floor. This is about improving our health, not about getting hurt. Please be careful. I mean it. Be careful.

Pulsating Hunger Pains that disappear and then re-emerge throughout the day. For some persons, hunger is monstrous in the morning. But for the vast majority, the hunger troll shows up mostly at night. In short, hunger will always be a part of our lives, and it is our task to master it rather than allow it to enslave us as it **CAN AND WILL** if we let it.

In my case, hunger was very strong in the first week to 10 days of intermittent fasting, and then I found myself getting used to always being 'a little' hungry. After a while, I loved it because I began to feel more alert, more energetic, optimistic... I slept better.

I actually **SLEPT THROUGH THE NIGHT** and woke up feeling terrific. Before the fast, I constantly woke up at night to urinate, or like a raving lunatic wanting to raid the fridge. After a while, I would go to sleep at 11PM, close my eyes and, when I opened them, it was 6AM!

For me, this was nothing less than a total miracle. And I felt great... refreshed and ready to go! All of that just from getting used to eating less and being a little hungry.

Much better than getting stuffed like a boar as I used to.

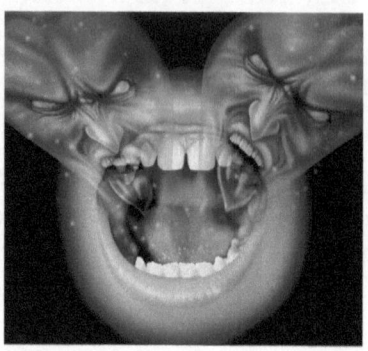

Bad Breath, Metallic Taste in Mouth, <u>White Sticky Film on Tongue</u> – These are all good indications that your body is eliminating toxicity.

Most of these symptoms pass after 14 days (*on average*).

For bad Breath, I suggest that you get sugarless mints and keep them handy until the process ends.

Metallic Taste In the Mouth usually means that there are excessive (*and toxic*) heavy metals accumulated in your system.

I recall having this constant sulfur and 'steel' taste in my mouth for about a week.

White Sticky Film on the Tongue can be disgusting, but it's a sign that the body is cleansing. For these symptoms, the best thing you can do is to keep drinking a lot of water.

Make sure to brush your teeth regularly. Keep a travel toothbrush with you if you spend a lot of time out. Mouthwash is also helpful.

Diarrhea or Constipation – All of the fecal matter adhered to your colon will either start gushing out in diarrhea or incite short-term constipation.

I know that this is disgusting, but it happens. If you have eaten poorly for a long time, or have simply abused sugar or fat, your body may respond to the water fast by starting to expel all of the toxic filth in this fashion.

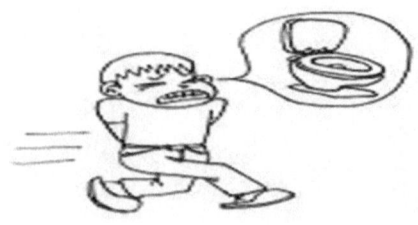

If **Diarrhea** Strikes, simply continue to follow the fast as outlined. Should it become severe, see your pharmacist and ask him or her for an over-the-counter recommendation.

Continue with the intermittent fast. Fasting is a shock to the body, but it will finally get the message and react favorably to what you are doing. If you have diarrhea, make sure to keep yourself hydrated.

Make it a point to drink at least one gallon of water daily. Stay close to a bathroom at all times. If you go out, make sure that you are always aware where the nearest restroom is. Seriously, you want to get to the toilet promptly anytime you need to.

If **Constipation** is The Case, visit your local pharmacy and ask your pharmacist about a stool softener. I personally use a herbal laxative called <u>Herbs & Prunes</u>. It works like a charm every time and is not harsh on my stomach. Take one tablet to start.

Do not exceed four tablets in one day. But do this only if you fail to eliminate anything for at least three days. Give your body enough time to do it on its own.

Irritability / Mood Swings – If you have ever seen The Flintstones, you may remember Fred walking around growling on the episode where he is placed on a diet.

Be prepared to be a little *"short-fused"* during this time fasting and cleansing.

Be aware that you will not be as patient as you normally would. Tell your loved ones not to take it personally if - initially - you are less social that what they are accustomed.

This is normal and will pass.

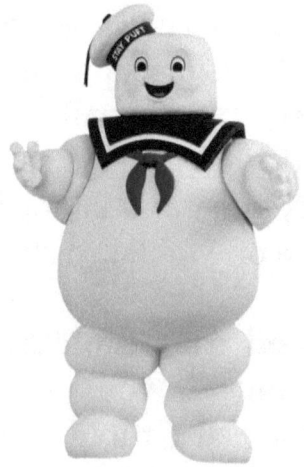

Facial Puffiness & Feeling Bloated – This symptom is much more marked for persons who consume large amounts of salt and/or sugar. I personally was bloated to the max like the **Stay Puft Marshmallow Man** (*pictured above*).

So being puffy was nothing new. I looked like somebody had stuck huge balloons on my cheeks. It was hideous.

Fasting took care of that and my face today is that of a normal human being rather than a cartoon character. That is a lot of symptoms, but rarely does **ONE** person experience them all. And remember, they will subside and mostly pass after approximately 14 days.

Continue to surrender to the process and stay put. Let the body do what it does best. Your body knows how to take care of you. Your body and digestive system thank you for this break.

Your body is loyal and noble ... it is unleashing amazing weight loss and healing power even as we speak. All you have to do is hang on and let the process run its course.

Chapter 9
Assignments

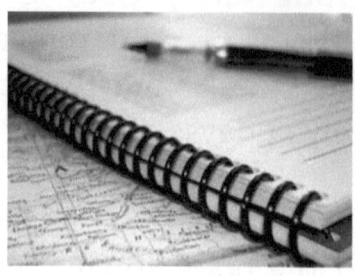

Purchase ALL of the Ingredients Needed to Complete the Entire 10-day Colon Cleanse. It will be much more beneficial to have all of the ingredients handy, so you can focus on the daily preparation and consumption, NOT on having to go out shopping because you forgot or did not get an ingredient. Seriously, step one is to get all of the ingredients... every single one of them. THEN you can come back home and start preparation

Drink the Colon Cleanse remedy for 10 days, strictly adhering to the banned foods we looked at earlier. When hunger and/or cravings come around to hassle you, drink two large glasses of water and breathe. Spend time writing about your health-related goals.

Fill your mind with the powerful reasons why you want to accomplish this detox cleanse, and in which way will your life be improved with total body detoxification.

The cost of this cleansing process is minimal in comparison to the huge health benefits that you will receive, not to mention added quality years of life!

Stay Close to and Communicate with at least one person that you trust who will support you in this task and not judge.

Any type of detox cleansing is initially going to be challenging, so it helps a lot to have someone standing by to give you a hand and cheer you on. So don't be a Lone Ranger please.

This step is designed to give you ongoing "human" support. Human support will prove invaluable to you during this cleanse. Go to Fitness Through Fasting's -- Fasting Forum and post messages. Ask for a buddy! Read other people's posts and reach out! You will find many others on the same path. You may even make life-long friends!

When tempted to stray, always remember: Nothing Tastes as Good as Thin Feels!

God bless and Godspeed,

ROBERT DAVE JOHNSTON

Grab The Entire Collection:

Volume 1: The 'Permanent Weight Loss' Diet

Volume 2: The Intermittent Fasting Weight Loss Formula

Volume 3: How to Lose 30 Pounds (Or More) In 30 Days with Juice Fasting

Volume 4: Lose The Belly Fat Fast, And For Good!

Volume 5: Lose the Emotional Baggage: Transform Your Mind & Spirit with Fasting

Volume 6: How to Break a Fast (or Diet) and Keep the Weight Off

Volume 7: Compilation Volumes 1-6 -> Get All 5 For The Price Of 3!

Also by Robert Dave Johnston:

How to Lose Weight & Keep it Off by Transforming the Mind & Behaviors

Volume 1: How to Build a Rock-Solid Foundation That Supports Long-Term Weight Loss

Volume 2: How to Lose Weight & Keep it Off By Reprogramming The Subconscious Mind

Volume 3: How to Beat Diet Hunger and Junk Food Cravings

Volume 4: How to Escape the Diet "Time Trap" and Succeed in Weight Loss

Volume 5: How to Cheat on Your Diet (And Get Away With It)

Volume 6, Compilation: All 5 for the Price Of 3

Also By Robert Dave Johnston:

Detoxify Your Body, Lose Weight, Get Healthy & Transform Your Life

Volume 1- The 10-Day 'At Home' Colon Cleansing Formula

Volume 2- The 30-Day Kidney, Parasite & Liver Detox Weight Loss Method

Volume 3- Lose Weight Fast & Detoxify With Intermittent Fasting & At-Home Coffee Enemas

Volume 4 - Compilation: Get All 3 For The Price Of 2! Detoxify Your Body, Lose Weight, Get Healthy & Transform Your Life - Volumes 1-3

Don't forget to check the articles and growing health community at: FitnessThroughFasting.com